LORETO SIXTH FORM COLLEGE

610·73

7 DAY
BOOK

GETTING INTO

Nursing and

Midwifery

JANET HIGGINS

D0318592

TROTMAN

This second edition published in 2001
by Trotman & Company Ltd
2 The Green, Richmond, Surrey TW9 1PL
First edition published 1996

© Trotman and Company Limited 2001

British Library Cataloguing in Publication Data
A catalogue record for this book is available from the British Library

ISBN 0 85660 547 6

All rights reserved. No part of this publication may be reproduced, stored in a
retrieval system or transmitted in any form or by any means, electronic and
mechanical, photocopying, recording or otherwise without prior permission of
Trotman and Company Ltd.

Typeset by Florence Production Ltd, Stoodleigh, Devon
Printed and bound in Great Britain by Creative Print & Design (Wales) Ltd

CONTENTS

About the author   v

Dedication   vi

Part 1 The scenario   1

1   Important beginnings   3

2   New developments in nursing and midwifery   7

3   How nursing and midwifery education
     reflects practice developments   14

4   New roles in nursing and midwifery: Where
     do I see myself in five years time?
     Case studies, people like you   22

5   What do I have to offer, and what should
     I study before I apply?   36

6   Necessary personal attributes for a career as
     a nurse or midwife   43

7   How will these personal attributes be
     assessed?   45

8   Some notes on higher education   49

9   The effect of NHS policy changes on
     getting into nursing and midwifery   53

**Part 2 Essential preparations for a successful
outcome**   57

10   OK, so I still want to be a nurse   59

Contents

11 Applying through the system   61

12 Choosing your college or university
    and getting chosen   64

13 If at first you don't succeed . . .   67

14 I am a registered nurse and wish to study
    for a degree   68

Part 3 Next steps in lifelong learning   71

15 Personal record of education and
    professional practice (PREP)   73

16 I have a diploma in nursing or midwifery
    and wish to study for a degree   74

17 The professional bodies   76

18 Resource information and contact data   78

ABOUT THE AUTHOR

Janet Higgins has been involved with nurse education for many years. Following graduation at London University with a medical degree, MB, BS and an Intercalated Honours BSc in Physiology with Biochemistry, Janet started her career at the Royal Free Hospital School of Medicine, in medical research in the department of pharmacology. It was as a lecturer at the hospital, teaching medical students, that she was given the task of 'lecturing the nurses'. This was the start of a rewarding association with all the changes in nurse education that have happened since the 1970s to the present day.

Janet Higgins has held a number of senior posts, including senior lecturer at the University of Leicester Medical School, and principal lectureships at St Andrews Hospital School of Occupational Therapy (Northampton), and at Gloucestershire College of Arts and Technology (GlosCat). As head of School of Health and Social Care at GlosCat she was responsible for the education of social workers as well as community nurses. Here, too, she developed new courses for practice nurses, working together with the local GP practices, their supervisory health trusts, and the education officers of the English National Board for Nursing, Midwifery and Health Visiting.

Currently Janet Higgins is involved in developing health sciences interrelating with nursing, midwifery and health trust management at Middlesex University.

During her work there she has been involved with the validation of both degree and diploma programmes leading to professional qualifications in nursing. She was also appointed external examiner to the Royal College of Nursing Institute, and held similar appointments at Kingston University, and at Guildford College of Further and Higher Education for Health Studies for qualified nurses in practice.

The focus for this book would not have occurred without Tony Higgins, Chief Executive of the University and Colleges Admissions service (UCAS). As a consequence of this first-hand knowledge of the nursing education changes, national health policy changes, application procedures, and many, many students, this book seemed inevitable. Having been a successful part of the Trotman 'Getting into' series, the book has been substantially rewritten for its second edition to incorporate the many changes that have taken place in the short space of time since the book's inception.

DEDICATION

To nursing, a practice and philosophy that has formed a more central part of my life than I would have expected.

Janet Higgins
London January 2001

Part 1
THE SCENARIO

Chapter 1
IMPORTANT BEGINNINGS

So you want to be a nurse. Alternatively, or additionally, you want to care for expectant mothers and be involved in the successful birth of their offspring.

Roles within nursing and midwifery have always been changing, reflecting the dynamics and professional demands placed upon them. Social pressures, changing communities, technological changes, human values, Europeanisation and globalisation are all having their impact on the development of the way that nurses and midwives are employed, evaluated, work with others, are remunerated and valued.

It is a time of exciting change. The problem is the pace of change, sometimes too fast, sometimes infuriatingly slow. These same pressures may continue for some time, but the possibilities of real job satisfaction and challenge are emerging from these drivers for change. It is probably one of the most exciting times to join (or rejoin) the professions of nursing and midwifery.

People make the decision to enter nursing or midwifery education at various stages in their personal or career development. Some make the decision while studying for A-levels, or vocational A-levels, at school or further education college; others during the course of a university degree. Many enter nursing following work in other jobs or professions, entering as mature students, (ie aged 21 or over) with non-standard entry qualifications. Yet others, a new group, may in the future enter through being initially a nursing assistant employed by a hospital or community trust, developing educationally through the vocational qualifications done whilst associated with that employment.

The important thing is not to make up your mind to go into nursing or midwifery practice until you are ready. This book aims to give all those who wish to become nurses or midwives – at whatever stage – a practical approach to self-assessment, together with information and advice on the routes available.

All would-be nurses and midwives must have gathered sufficient recent and relevant information to make an informed choice, especially at this present time of change in the National Health Service (NHS) and in the number and variety of roles that can be achieved within nursing and midwifery in their widest contexts.

Getting into Nursing is written to try to make your choices easier and more effective. The aim is to assist you to make a simple checklist of questions and consider areas for discussion. Some of the key resources and sources of information referred to in the book are listed in the Bibliography, together with some useful addresses on pp 78–83.

Have you really identified that you wish to become a nurse or midwife, and know the reasons why you have made your choice, rather than choosing to enter one of the other caring or interventive professions such as those allied to medicine – occupational therapy or physiotherapy – or indeed medicine itself – dentistry – or one of the complementary therapies such as herbal medicine for example?

Whatever you do, make absolutely sure that you have gained enough information about the various caring professions and their educational requirements to be able to make an informed choice, not only for yourself but for those who will be supporting and developing your choice. You are very likely to have to talk about these matters at interview in order to gain a place in the university or college to which you have chosen to apply.

If you are uncertain of your career in health or health care, then you might well be advised to study the wider relevant subjects covered within a modular degree in Health Studies or Health Sciences. When you have clarified your overall career plan, you could then enter your chosen clinical career, with confidence that you have made the right choice.

You may choose to study for a Diploma in Nursing or Diploma in Midwifery to supplement the degree that you have already achieved. The real question you have to ask yourself is 'Have I sufficient personal resources to stand the exciting pace of change when linked to new and demanding professional responsibilities?' This applies to almost all the clinical professions, but most especially to nursing and midwifery today.

If you are a little further along this road of discovery, the self-analysis explored in Part 1 will give you the confidence to apply for and be successful in the next steps of lifelong learning. Chapters 15–18 have been written with this in mind. Exciting professional work is constantly updated, making practice relevant to the changing needs of society. So it is with nursing and midwifery, both of which require you to look to the future and ask 'What will I be doing in five years' time, and what preparations do I need to make to get there, or to make my practice better?' This is as true for those already qualified and in practice as it is for the novice.

It is likely that much greater resources will be made available by government for the NHS to develop the areas of responsibility of the 'nurse practitioner', including that of prescribing and administering drugs appropriate for clinical intervention and care. Politically within the clinical professions there will be a marked change in clinical responsibility towards the lead-role of the nurse and midwife. Included in the resources listed at the end of the book is a reference to the NHS web site that outlines the new policy developments in this context.

The rewards of patient care, both direct and indirect, are considerable. Occasionally there is sadness, and often there is a small dose of politics but, as they say, all human life is there, and you could be an active and highly relevant part of it.

The professional focus of the nurse or midwife has always been the care of the whole person. For the midwife there is the added bonus of two people, the mother and the child. This philosophy is still central to the continuing and future roles of nurses and midwives during times of development and change.

Other professions have other focuses and philosophies. The main professional focus of a medical practitioner is different to that of a nurse. He or she is concerned primarily with what is causing the person to be unwell, or why they have the symptoms they are complaining about. The doctor is concerned to make a specific diagnosis in order to improve the health or the condition of the patient. The nurse is primarily concerned with the patient, their comfort and their care. It is easy to see how the two roles are complementary. Health education and health promotion are areas shared by both professions, but approached from different perspectives.

The professional philosophies of both professions are central to what a nurse may have to take account of when, later in the career progression, he or she may wish to consider new government education initiatives that may offer some suitably experienced nurses the opportunity to become doctors, by fast-track courses within combined medical and nursing university hospital education units.

Chapter 2
NEW DEVELOPMENTS IN NURSING AND MIDWIFERY

DAUGHTERS OF FLORENCE

Until recently very little appeared to have changed in the public's romantic image of the pretty young nurse in the starched white uniform at the bedside of the sick or injured person. In one notable London hospital student nurses were still called Nightingales, and were trained with a thoroughness that only the 'lady with the lamp' herself could have exceeded. However, there can be no doubt that her pioneering style would have led that same lady to be at the forefront of the professional and educational developments in nursing today. One of these key educational developments, 'Project 2000', has had, and will continue to have considerable professional benefits and consequences.

PROJECT 2000

Project 2000 was the name given to the recent profound changes and developments in nurse education, designed and implemented originally to meet the challenges of the 21st century. A fuller account of these innovative educational programmes is given in Chapter 3. To understand the real relevance of these courses and to assist you in any discussion you may have with those close to you, during the application process or at interview, you should read this chapter.

The fundamental review of nursing education represented by Project 2000 was undertaken about 15 years ago, spearheaded by the leaders of the profession and the nursing professional bodies. Its purpose was to

7

bring nurses to graduate level of education, and to allow them to work alongside other health professions, notably medicine, with equivalent professional recognition, where their contribution would be appropriately recognised and rewarded. The programme was delayed by a variety of inter-professional and political issues, not least of which was the unavailability of funding to free up unqualified nurses from work rosters in order to take time for in-depth learning – at the bedside, in the clinic and also within university and college environments – to develop knowledge, skills and attitudes to a level that reflects the demands placed upon the professional practitioner.

The national boards for Nursing, Midwifery and Health Visiting were largely responsible for the initiation and early implementation of these educational changes, together with the colleges and institutions of higher education (including the former polytechnics, now the 'new' universities), which formed constituent partners in the process. Publications outlining many of these new developments are available from the NHS Careers office, the address of which appears at the end of this book.

Nursing and midwifery education proceeding to professional registration for practice is now exclusively via the model brought about in Project 2000, by means of the Diploma of Higher Education (DipHE) in Nursing or Midwifery Studies, and direct entry degree studies in nursing and midwifery, in colleges of higher education and universities, in partnership with clinical agencies, hospital and community trusts.

It is important to note that nursing and midwifery can now be studied by two separate routes. You no longer have to study nursing and qualify as a nurse before you undertake midwifery studies. You may enter midwifery by direct entry for either DipHE or degree studies. Degrees may be either single subject, or joint honours by top-up study from the Diploma. It is also possible to undertake a Masters Degree in Midwifery studies, but you will need to gain initial qualification to practise via diploma or degree routes, and the entry criteria are strictly regulated in this context. You can find details of Masters programmes via the ECCTIS database and web site (see page 82), and from individual university and college prospectuses.

Diploma and undergraduate degree qualifications both lead to professional qualification, and entry to the first part of the professional register. However there are some differences, and these stem largely from the minimum entry qualifications required for each course and level to be studied (generally one A-level or equivalent for the DipHE, and two A-levels or equivalent for the degree) that satisfy the educational institutes' requirements. In addition there are some very important professional minimum entry requirements that are common to both the degree and diploma – these are largely involved with professional practice, and clarified in Chapter 5.

Diploma and degree students usually receive monies from different primary sources in order to support their studies, but there is some overlap in bursary provision, if this has been sponsored and supported by the local hospital trusts. Degree students generally receive their money via the usual local education authority student loan system, and the diploma student via a bursary from the Department of Health that is organised and administered by the college or university at which the place for study has been gained and accepted. The Department of Health bursaries are related to the resource allocation identified for each region to educate and train a limited number of nurses and midwives for that region, related to staffing needs.

The programmes of both diploma and degree studies comprise an initial period of prolonged study, the Common Foundation Programme (CFP), which develops core areas of nursing studies common to all the later branch programmes: adult, mental health, child, and learning disability nursing.

As stated previously, midwifery is studied as an independent programme, pursuing the same educational principles, to degree and diploma (DipHE), within universities and colleges of higher education, in partnership with hospital and community care trusts.

Other specialisms, which also earlier followed post-registration nursing certificate routes, such as health visiting, community nursing, school nurse, occupational health nurse and practice nurse, continue to form further specialist career pathways, and still depend on initial registration to practise.

During the early years of the health reforms, in the mid-1980s, the job description of each nursing appointment was analysed into a portfolio of skill mixes. Jobs and remuneration were reviewed to allow senior nurses to achieve better and more efficient use of their time, supported by junior or assistant colleagues undertaking the less difficult skilled areas of the 'job'. Nurses were thereby graded A–I for appropriate skills designated to their appointment and remunerated accordingly.

A Grade A nurse may receive £9000–£11010, rising to a Grade I nurse earning £25,770–£29,205 for a basic working week of 37½ hours. Nursing care is provided over 24 hours, seven days a week, and consequently there is also a small allowance made for night shifts and weekends, which may increase salaries by an extra 10 per cent. There is also an additional allowance for working in London (see NHS Careers' Pay Information Leaflet 2000).

Pay grades apply to skill mixes for hospital, community and GP practice employment. Nurses in the NHS have five weeks (25 working days) holiday a year, together with additions for bank holidays and statutory days with days off in lieu, if they are worked.

Government is working towards higher remuneration for higher levels of responsibility, as in the role of the nurse consultant, which may ultimately reach £40,000. Similar appointments to senior roles in hospital and community trusts will reach similar levels of remuneration.

Further details about career choices and developments can be found in Chapter 4. You should read this if you are thinking of entering one of the many specialisms, especially if you already hold a degree, or a Diploma in Nursing Studies that you may consider converting to a degree, in either Health Studies, Nursing Studies, or one of the many joint honours combinations. These are available both in skills-based learning and in underlying theoretical studies, as listed on the UCAS web site. It is also worthwhile exploring some of the postgraduate prospectuses published by individual universities and colleges or through the ECCTIS database.

Since this whole educational and inter-professional area is developing very rapidly, it is always worth checking these things out for yourself. The UCAS web site and UCAS *Handbook* apply to undergraduate courses only.

Postgraduate courses listings are available on the ECCTIS database and in a handbook, *Graduate Courses*, published separately.

Do make sure that you check the date of the information on any web site as its usefulness is only as good as its 'updatedness'. Individual universities and colleges also publish their own postgraduate prospectuses, as well as having their own individual web sites – check these as well.

PROFESSIONAL COLLEAGUES

As government policy, or social policy as it is termed, has indirectly assisted the new developments in the education of nurses to meet the challenges that they will face in the new millennium, then it is important to mention some other professionals with whom nurses and midwives will work either directly or indirectly, and alongside whom nurses and midwives may occasionally work in educational programmes during undergraduate studies. This area involves social workers and others who are involved in community care. It also involves shared learning within degree programmes together with medical or dental students in some institutions, and sometimes occupational therapists and physiotherapists.

Social workers, like nurses, are educated to diploma, degree and postgraduate levels of education. A common area of education focus with nursing is that of learning disability, one of the branch programmes in the model of Project 2000. The Community Care Act 1990 is but slowly working its way towards changing the balance of care away from confining institutions and into the wider community. This frequently seems an uphill task to all those involved. However the primary changes have already taken place, with the subsequent alignment of practice studies and placements in education.

PRIMARY HEALTH CARE AND PRACTICE NURSES

(See Angelina and Jackie in Case Studies in Chapter 4, pages 26 and 31.)

Before the NHS social policy changes got underway, following enactment in 1990, qualified nurses began to be employed more fully and more frequently in health centres in general practice, as practice nurses, working alongside general practitioners and other members of the primary health care team. Many, with full registration (the then Registered General Nurses, RGNs) worked with full autonomy whilst being responsible to the general practitioner. Others, State Enrolled Nurses (SENs), could only work under supervision of an RGN. SENs have subsequently been required to undertake conversion courses, validated by the four national boards of Nursing, Health Visiting and Midwifery, to develop their education skills to Registration Certification (see Chapter 15) and others have undertaken the three or four years of full-time study to achieve an undergraduate degree in Nursing Studies, following entry to university as mature students.

CARE ASSISTANT COLLEAGUES

(See Jo in Case Studies in Chapter 4, page 32.)

Unregistered individuals, care assistants, nursing assistants, or helpers, may assist with hospital bedside care as part of their job specification, with defined tasks under supervision. However people in these jobs are not usually on recognised programmes of study leading to nursing or other professional qualifications, and are not bound by professional codes of conduct – they rely on those provided by their nursing colleagues as supervisors.

Such care assistants, through their employment, may undertake a National Vocational Qualification (NVQ) which, by national recognition and standard, may be used for progression in learning and professional development. At a later time they may wish to be considered for entry as mature students to advanced programmes of study.

For entry to nursing or midwifery minimum entry requirements have to be met, and these are laid out in Chapter 5. Similarly regulation of professional conduct is primarily through the terms of their working contract. Vocational subjects' assessments being developed with post-16 studies thoughout the UK will be helpful to working nurse/care assistants as their own NVQ-assessed skills should become part of this assessed portfolio, and count towards the potential undergraduate application to nursing and midwifery studies programmes.

SUMMARY OF CHANGE

First, nursing and midwifery are at the centre of a health revolution. (See Sinead, Frances, Anita, Christopher and John in the case studies in Chapter 4.)

Second, how the government spends its money in keeping the nation well is largely changing from hospital bed to community care. The balance between the two modes is still being adjusted.

Third, the nurse is still very much the professional nurse. He or she, through professional and educational developments, will be able to contribute more effectively within these changing contexts. The Code of Professional Conduct of the United Kingdom Central Council for Nursing, Midwifery and Health Visiting (UKCC) shows how relevant the clinical and professional values and standards of the profession remain today. Nursing professionals are still and always will be accountable for their own practice and responsible for the nursing needs of their patients and clients.

Fourth, the autonomy of both nursing and midwifery has increased substantially, by being underwritten by government policy (see NHS Careers literature, at the end of this book).

Chapter 3
HOW NURSING AND MIDWIFERY EDUCATION REFLECTS PRACTICE DEVELOPMENTS

Many of the changes now taking place in nurse and midwifery education have been determined by changes in society.

Life expectancy has considerably improved in the UK and the western world, with increasing improvement in housing and diet and the development of life-preserving drugs. Meanwhile, birth rate is declining, thus altering the demographic profile of the population. There are more older people, who are expected to place greater demands on the health care system whether they are ill or not. In addition babies who might have been stillborn in earlier times are saved by skilled and possibly high-tech care. Other less vulnerable babies, all of whom might have been born in hospital a decade ago, are now born in low-tech, home-from-home units, assisted by midwives, working both in the hospital and in the community.

The Department of Health set targets to improve the health of the nation by the year 2000 and beyond, which creates an increased emphasis on health education and preventive measures to improve community health, and further to improve care in the community.

People as patients and clients must be cared for as individuals, and it is important for nurses, along with other members of the health care team, to understand a person's background and circumstances that affect his or her health in their day-to-day environment if they are to help individuals achieve lasting health.

A body of recent research has shown that those individuals who take an active role in their care tend to get better more quickly. Listening and explaining in the caring context are therefore significant components of effective practice, enabling patients and clients to achieve this. Research has also indicated that patients undergoing day-case surgery may recover more quickly than their counterparts in hospital environmental care during the recovery period. A patient's home environment appears to be more conducive to recovery of health than the pressures associated with staying in a hospital ward. These research papers can be found in recent editions of the *British Medical Journal* (*BMJ*) at www.bmj.com.

These major areas of research focus on some of the fundamental changes that have been taking place recently in nursing and nursing care. Working in multiprofessional teams, or independently with autonomy and responsibility, is now the order and challenge of the day. Consequently these are very exciting times for you to be considering entering into or developing within the nursing and midwifery professions.

PROJECT 2000 – A MILESTONE ON THE WAY

General style and content of the model

Project 2000 is the core programme for nurse education today, and it is the fundamental pattern of education for nurses and midwives to undertake in order to register to practise. This holds true whether study is towards a diploma or an honours degree in undergraduate studies. The name of the project, whilst still acknowledged, is moving into the background as time passes and further developments are superimposed on the original template.

There are differences in the various courses offered at different institutions, but they all uphold, by their initial validations, the central themes and structure of Project 2000. Each course fulfils all the educational requirements needed in order to practise, and fulfils the practice requirements of the UKCC, by agreement with the partners at validation, including the hospital trusts and the university or college at which the course is held. Different institutions have adapted the core frameworks to reflect their strengths in staff expertise in special interests and excellence.

It is therefore highly relevant for you to find out from university and college prospectuses, and from visits to open days, what the different strengths of each course are. The quality of each course has been regularly assessed by many authorities, including assessment that takes place at its initial validation.

The Universities Higher Education Quality Assurance Agency (QAA) also rates the areas of programmes within the particular university context, out of 24 points. Those with 22 or above rank as 'Excellent'. Universities or colleges with a lower rating in their areas of programmes may just cause you to ask why, and how long ago the rating was given. You may find that the area of concern has now been greatly improved, or it was a matter that was not going to affect your course and studies anyway. University rankings are fashionable, but this is only one of many assessments of their virtues. You as the prospective student and applicant may have other views.

The major choice that you have to make is which of these courses' approaches, strengths, locations and facilities best suits your own interests, needs and aptitudes. Remember, you will be studying there for a minimum of three years, possibly four, during initial qualification.

The core programme

The core programme is made up of two main parts: the Common Foundation Programme (CFP), and the Branch Programme (BP).

The CFP allows you to develop your knowledge of people systematically, from studies in psychology and sociology (the family and community), together with biology, or life sciences. These studies, and core skills (such as communication skills), take place in parallel with those in nursing studies, both theory and early practice.

At this stage you will be supernumerary, ie over and above the workforce numbers when you are learning in a clinical setting. This may be in the community or in a hospital placement, and is usually rotated to give you a wide variety of experience. As your experience builds you will start to apply your broad base of knowledge to an individual patient in his or her circumstances. The CFP allows you to experience placements in the different branch programme areas. You will probably have already made your choice of branch programme, but you may find that there is room for a change of mind.

Throughout the programme there is an increasing thread of development towards understanding effective use of human resources, together with a knowledge of financial accountability. This may sound a little difficult to comprehend at application time, but it simply means that the nurse or midwife is now a manager in the widest sense, whether leading a nursing team, handling resource allocation for a unit or developing new approaches to care.

The branch programme you undertake, which will depend on your initial choice and the availability of places, will form the second part of the programme, taking a further 18 months of the total three years, either as a diploma or degree programme. The branch programmes are: adult nursing, mental health nursing, learning disability nursing, children's nursing.

Although you will have been supernumerary in the earlier part of the course, you will now move on to learn through 1000 hours of rostered service, making an important contribution to the nursing team, and learning through the implications of practice and accountability.

Some institutions may offer all the branch programmes, others may offer only two or three from the options available. Not all courses are alike. Make sure you obtain the current prospectus for the courses in question. Many of the institutions in which the courses are set are undergoing considerable reorganisation and development.

It possible to 'top up' the diploma course or extend studies to honours degree via further study at Level 3 (see pages 50–51 for an explanation of this term), undertaking health studies, midwifery studies or nursing studies designed to achieve this. The combinations of subjects have developed over time, and by consulting the UCAS web site you will find a treat in store when you discover what the range of options open to you are, and the variety of institutions offering these, either as single honours or as joint honours degree top-up programmes.

These studies allow the student to assess critically the subject that he or she is studying. The work may also build on the initial study of research method that will be part of the diploma course.

You may also have to undertake a research project, possibly within a clinical area or on a topic related to practice.

Course locations

Almost all diploma and degree studies in clinical subjects are officially sited on university and college of higher education campuses, then range through various hospital and community locations during clinical studies. This allows you to have all the benefits of a university campus life, mixing with many people studying a variety of subjects, and also to have your own specialist areas focused for you to attain practice and theory competence to gain qualification in your chosen field and career.

Always try to enquire about clinical areas and where they may be when you visit the various campuses, and enquire about these aspects at open day or, at the very latest, at your interview.

Course titles

Degrees are usually awarded at honours level, sometimes as a BA (Hons) and sometimes as a BSc (Hons), depending on the overall sciences, social sciences or humanities content of the programmes. As nursing practice is moving towards prescribing, the majority of these programmes now lead to the award of a BSc. The subject combinations offered as the top up to a diploma in either nursing or midwifery may affect whether you are awarded an Honours BA or an Honours BSc, as the final classification of any degree is largely based on the quality of attainment in the final year, and at Level 3 studies. A fuller description of levels of undergraduate studies is given on pages 50–51.

Course length

Courses tend to vary in length from three to four years full time, and both honours degree courses and diploma courses may take three years. You may like to ask whether the normal student term or the semester system applies to the course you are interested in, as you may need to use the long vacation for rostered hours of service or for observations and placement studies. Loans and bursaries are normally adjusted to support these commitments, but you need to know what the pressures may be *before* you enter a particular course, rather than once you are on it.

Entry requirements

Statutory requirements

Entry requirements may vary slightly from institution to institution, depending on the variation in overall content planned for the course, but there are certain minimum subject passes that have to be achieved in order to fulfil statutory (or legal) requirements to enter nursing and, slightly differently, midwifery.

To study nursing you must have a minimum of five subject passes at GCSE or equivalent.

To study midwifery the five subject passes must include a science subject (eg biology) and also either English language or literature.

You must be at least 17 and a half years of age on entry, but you are allowed to apply at 16.

University and college educational requirements

Until September 2002 the minimum entry requirement to study for the DipHE is one good A-level GCE pass, or its equivalent, and four other subjects studied to GCSE pass level, or equivalent, together with many other personal attributes that can be assessed at interview or written about in the references concerning you.

The minimum entry requirements to study for an honours degree is two good A-level passes, together with three other subjects to GCSE pass standard or equivalent. Other (highly important) attributes will be assessed at interview together with your referees' information about these.

Mature students may enter without the formal qualifications quoted above, but need to demonstrate prior and recent learning in five subject areas, or the equivalent, thereby fulfilling the statutory or legal requirements listed. This may be achieved by completing a year studying on an Access to Nursing Course. This certification is accepted for entry to nursing and midwifery providing that the additional statutory requirements are met.

Most local further education colleges run these programmes, both to prepare the student for study in higher education and to test and develop the beginnings of clinical awareness in the student in the group situation of the course setting. These courses also allow you to undertake other units of study similar to those taken by post-16 students at school. You will need to enquire about what could be on offer for you, as each programme is likely to differ owing to the level of demand each college has for each unit of study, as well as the facilities it is able to offer. You have everything to gain by asking questions.

Most universities will be interested in what earlier experience and qualifications (formal or informal) you bring to the programme. Some will allow you to offer these as certificated evidence of sufficient earlier equivalent studies in the areas required, as in earlier NVQs. Clearly some of these are somewhat formal statutory requirements that have to be met. Popular universities and programmes can be choosy, and as a consequence there is an element of competition. To assist in finding out about specific courses' unwritten requirements and styles, see Heap, 2000.

September 2000 saw the start of the new post-16 curriculum (known as Curriculum 2000) in schools and colleges.

These changes involve major revisions to GCE A-levels and the introduction of the new Advanced Subsidiary (AS), replacing AGNVQ by Vocational A-levels (6 and 12 unit), and vocational Advanced Subsidiary (VAS), with opportunities to provide evidence of key skills in all post-16 programmes of study (eg the new key skills qualification).

When students apply to higher education institutions with many different styles of qualifying certificates it is often difficult for admissions tutors to make comparisons between individual students' achievements. Recently UCAS has developed a framework that should assist the comparison of certificated achievement which applicants to higher education present to their chosen universities or colleges. The UCAS tariff within the NVQ framework will also give numerical equivalence between qualifications in different parts of the UK, eg Scotland and England. You can find out more on this by visiting the UCAS web site. All students applying for September 2002 entry to higher education will have to apply using this new UCAS tariff.

For mature entry students there will be support and development in the key skills areas by study modules inserted into all degree and diploma programmes. This means that all students on higher education courses from 2002 will be able to demonstrate that by the end of the first year of their studies in higher education they will have the listed number of key skills and will be on an equal footing with the students entering from schools.

Chapter 4
NEW ROLES IN NURSING AND MIDWIFERY: WHERE DO I SEE MYSELF IN FIVE YEARS TIME? CASE STUDIES PEOPLE LIKE YOU

HANDS-ON CARE

You will have discovered from Chapter 3 that it is currently possible to qualify as a nurse or a midwife either at diploma (DipHE) or honours degree level, studying for three, three and a half or four years depending on your course. The earliest age at which you may start is 17½, but the upper limit on age for entry is less easy to define, and depends on guidelines from each institution among other things.

Throughout the UK, and within several regions including Scotland and Northern Ireland, there are currently 401 advertised programmes in nursing in universities and colleges. Some of these courses may allow you to study nursing with another specialist subject after you have gained your DipHE, and lead on to graduation with an honours degree.

Again, at time of going to press, there are 41 listed programmes for midwifery, some as pre-registration, some as post-registration (eg as nursing and midwifery), or as midwifery studies. Some programmes can be undertaken as 'shortened courses' by accreditation of prior learning (APL) by the university or college which accepts you. You may study midwifery as a single subject throughout your studies, but there are also programmes available to study midwifery with another subject after the diploma, when topping up to the honours degree, such as with community studies, health visiting, public health, health management, health sciences or disability. Complementary therapies may ultimately be included in this group as well. Again it would be worthwhile for you to check the up-to-date listings on the UCAS web site, as well as the universities web page on the NHS Careers site.

A few programmes, mostly nursing, or post-registration top up, are available for a February start, as well as for the usual September start. It is advisable to check the UCAS web site, and then directly with the university/college about the timing of entry, and the programme you have chosen.

Students may specialise through branch programmes to qualify for:

- adult nursing
- mental health nursing
- children's nursing
- learning disability nursing
- midwifery.

Prescribing for nursing and midwifery practice

Developments are under way to provide sufficient suitably educated and qualified nurses to take on the role of a prescribing practitioner. Current education for nurses and midwives is beginning to enlarge the area of study into pharmacology for prescribing for this purpose, in order that they may be able to prescribe medications in given circumstances.

Nurse-practitioner

Nurse-practitioner is the name given to an individual who has undergone a more intensive education in nursing, management and treatment practice following initial qualification, and who will largely work autonomously in the care of their patients. Such nurses are already thus qualified in New Zealand and the USA, and further developments in the UK are in progress, notably at institutes of advanced or postgraduate nursing studies.

NHS Call Direct Service

Also already on stream in the UK are the exciting initiatives involved within the 24-hour national telephone call service, NHS Call Direct, where telephone enquiries by patients are received by teams of senior nurses who advise on treatment in the short and medium term. They are supported in this role by computer data available to them as they advise the caller. Some of the advice may concern medication that may involve over the counter purchases or further medication prescription from a general practitioner, or in an emergency, via hospital casualty. (See Jennie in the case studies at the end of this chapter.)

A medical practitioner role?

New initiatives by government outline plans for suitably qualified and registered nurses to develop into independent medical care as medical practitioners, by further university and clinical training. These initiatives are focused on producing more doctors from nurses and involve a change in professional philosophy.

ONE STAGE BACK FROM HANDS-ON CARE?

Teaching and tutoring roles in nursing and midwifery practice

You may wish to consider the area of tutoring or even becoming a lecturer in nurse or midwifery education once you have achieved your early goals in clinical practice. Or you may want to pursue research in either of these fields by taking up a post at university. It is certainly an area of influence, either to develop practice or influence policy in health care. Most people in these roles retain their clinical, community or practitioner links in some context. It is seldom an either-or situation in professional choices. A new role is that of lecturer-practitioner. Most lecturers are required by their employment contract to have been in recent practice in some form.

The world is your oyster

You may wish to be able to influence a range of areas that affect nursing, midwifery, education or care directly or indirectly, but not necessarily have a direct hands-on role yourself at that time. Nurses and midwives are now well qualified to take on more senior and wider ranging roles in unit or trust management, either in a care team, unit or trust board role. The operational management of a hospital, for example, is likely to have a director of quality, incorporating the work of director of nursing, who will also have a seat on the full trust board.

Boards of trust management are responsible for community care as well as hospital care, the former in primary care, the latter largely in secondary care. Primary care, for those of you not familiar with the term, is the first point of contact for the patient or client. Treatment or advice may be given in the primary care setting, GP practice or community health centre. However the patient may be referred to a hospital or specialist clinic to receive secondary care, which may for example be an operation. Patients can sometimes be re-referred to a more central or specialist unit. This is termed tertiary care. Nurses are and will be more frequently involved throughout the whole structure of these new arrangements. Individually they may be responsible for assessing the health needs of the community, or managing resources to affect the care of a hospital ward, as the nursing sister and ward manager.

You may also ultimately wish to safeguard the areas of practice and professional standards, or influence government policy, and social policy, by working in or with one of the several professional nursing bodies such as the Royal College of Nursing and the Royal College of Midwifery. Again this is one further branch of nursing that could be open to you in due time and with committment, drive and personal and professional development. As a nurse, midwife or community nurse it is possible to enter politics to offer much of relevance in this currently disturbed world, either within a national organisation, in government or in an international organisation, working for the international agencies – Red Cross, World Health Organisation, British Council, Médicin Sans Frontières, United Nations to name a few.

CASE STUDIES OF PEOPLE ENTERING NURSING AND MIDWIFERY, 1998–2000

Names have been amended to preserve people's anonymity and confidentiality.

CAREER CHOICE OF PRACTICE NURSE

Angelina felt unable to achieve good results in the GCSE exams in the large classes in her inner city school. But since she had always wanted to become a nurse her school tutors advised her to join a smaller, more focused group studying an Advanced GNVQ Social Care programme over two years, until she was 19. She achieved a Merit profile. The programme included placement studies and course work based on the placements, and in community nursing. Angelina felt drawn to the work of the practice nurses at the nearby GP surgery/health centre where at least two GP practices were based, with 11 doctors and five practice nurses working in two groups. She noticed that several other health professions worked with the practice but were not employed by them directly.

Angelina liked the idea of working in a team whilst having key responsibility for special tasks that previously a doctor would do, such as taking blood pressures, blood samples for tests, and attending to minor injuries, but also new work such as regular surveys and running the well-man or well-woman clinics. One practice nurse ran an asthma clinic after taking further specialist courses during her work time.

Angelina applied for funding for her next steps in education and training via the NHS Students Grants Unit following her application to UCAS/NMAS to enter a diploma programme in nursing. She chose to enter the adult branch, and, from the information given on the UCAS web pages, found a suitable university not too far from her home where she could enter in the February cohort.

After finishing the AGNVQ in June, and receiving the results in September, Angelina spent five months working as a store assistant, and a month on holiday visiting her grandparents in a warm climate, as she felt the required commitment to her course might not allow such freedom in the next three years of study.

Although she gained a bursary for her studies she found that the money she had saved whilst working kept her out of immediate debt, and later she bought a low-cost computer to assist with her written assignments.

CAREER CHOICE OF MENTAL HEALTH NURSING

John left school in June with two A-level GCE passes, grades D and E, in theatre studies and psychology. His GCSE grades in six subjects, including maths and English language, were Bs and Cs. He was not quite sure what he wanted to do, nor where, at the time his school was advising him to fill in forms for the next stages of his education at university. He attended a careers fair and nursing seemed to be a reasonable career choice, as at least he could expect to have a job at the end of his studies, which might not be the case if he read psychology.

John's UCAS/NMAS application was for diploma studies in nursing, for the adult branch. However by the time he had had several interviews and done a little more homework on the subject he found his real interest lay in mental health nursing, as it had for many other young men before him. Another thing that confirmed his choice was that he had made two good friends who were going into the mental health branch following the Common Foundation Programme and it seemed much more the sort of challenge he wanted in his career choice. Also, from what his friends told him, it seemed he could achieve more in terms of career advancement. He discovered that mental health nurses are likely to work as members of a team, together with GPs, psychiatrists and social workers. In general, mental health nurses help plan the care and treatment for those who have mental illness. John was surprised to learn how frequently mental illness occurs and how most people are treated or cared for in the community. Everyone is treated as an individual, with their treatment tailored to their individual needs, and only occasionally returning to hospital when necessary. John worried a little about the difficulties that might occur if he was confronted with violence from his patients, but is now reassured that this is a rare occurrence and about as frequent as in any other branch of nursing.

John, being a 'groupy', was happy to learn that men are entering the nursing professional branches in increasing numbers year on year, now 10–11 per cent, with the mental health and learning disability branches heading the list. Also, with his mind on a more formal career pattern, he was pleased to learn that men tend to get promoted, in general, earlier than women. However he learned that this is due to many factors, not least of which is part-time working for female nurses possibly taking career breaks for family reasons. John is not married at the moment, but he does not rule out part-time working for himself in due course, as he thinks he would like to take an equal share in the care of any family he may have in the future. John has now entered university studying on a diploma programme, and having completed the 18 months of the Common Foundation Programme has just started on the branch leading to registration as a mental health nurse. He is very happy with both his programme and career choice as well as the university he is attending.

CAREER CHOICE OF CHILDREN'S NURSING

Frances, aged 25, lives in London near to her mother who works in a college. Frances has always wanted to work with children and had pinned her hopes on getting into primary school teaching, but she had difficulty in taking and passing mathematics in her GCSE examination, although she has passed seven other GCSE or equivalent CSE grades, including English language, some years ago. After several attempts to enter primary education courses she eventually settled for working in a bookshop as a sales assistant. Some of the work involved financial and other accounting.

When she was 22 her mother's friends told her that she could enter university as a mature student, where her life experiences might be taken more fully into account, that she would receive an interview to check these out, and that formal certificated GCE examinations could be waived for her entry. This was in early September, and Frances visited several local 'new' universities, but was still unable to get into primary education as all the programmes were full. She joined a joint honours degree programme in Health Studies, combined with Education Studies, obtaining (a then) grant from her local authority to study full time. Some of the study areas, or modules, in Education Studies involved learning about and working with children with learning difficulties.

The Health Studies modules took Frances into the world of the new thinking in the NHS, and the possibility of undertaking a module of study where a new career role may be explored through role-shadow, with follow-up analysis in tutorial groupwork. Children's nursing was a clear choice for Frances, which was reinforced by the role-shadow analysis.

The content of the modular Health Studies programme (which Frances achieved at a lower second honours classification) was sufficiently science based and mathematically skills oriented to be credited against her lack of GCSE mathematics at an earlier stage, to allow her to apply for and gain a place on an accelerated diploma programme in children's nursing over two years at a London university and associated hospitals. It was quite a pressurised time working over a shortened period, full time, for which Frances had a bursary on which to live, sometimes in hospital accommodation.

Frances has now completed her studies and is happily working as a full-time children's nurse, mostly within a hospital setting. Occasionally she goes out into the community to arrange for treatment or care for sick children from the hospital being cared for within their own homes, working with other professionals from the GP practice as well as the child's parents in terms of care planning and implementation. She works both in a team and independently and feels that she is trusted with a great deal of responsibility. She enjoys her life and receives much job satisfaction.

CAREER CHOICE OF LEARNING DISABILITY NURSING

Christopher, aged 32, initially wanted to work with children. However by taking on a summer job as an assistant in a summer camp working particularly with people with learning difficulties, including Down's syndrome, he discovered a new and rewarding world that he felt he wanted to contribute more to. At his local careers office, which he attended by appointment, he learned that the most suitable career path would be to train in nursing in the branch programme working with people with learning difficulties. There is some overlap with other professionals, for example social workers, but with the assistance of the careers counsellor Christopher decided that his approach would be through the diploma programme leading to registration in nursing for people with learning disabilities.

Christopher had formal certificated qualification of six CSEs, most at level 2 and 3, none at level 1, but including English, maths and French studies. However since the time he left school at 16 he has travelled quite widely and read a great deal. He tends to read all the main parts of a Sunday broadsheet newspaper most weekends. He worked for several years as an assistant technical manager in a photographic shop.

Two options were then open to Christopher to allow him to get into the university and community programmes of his choice, gleaned from the information available in books and discussions at his local careers office. Christopher could have his current knowledge and aptitudes tested to see if he could enter the programme at the first available opportunity or, alternatively, he could apply for either a recognised full-time or part-time Access to Nursing course at his local further education college, whilst still keeping on his job, if his manager agreed.

Christopher felt that the local Access course was rather wider than the area he wished to enter, and also worried about the pressure this might put him under at work. So through UCAS/NMAS he applied to enter his chosen programme at the main time in September, and requested through the university that he take a single-sitting test of core abilities, equal to about five GCSEs, known as the DC Test, and validated by the UKCC.

In Christopher's case it was the appropriate option, with his education being achieved after schooling over a number of years, from the foundation of the CSEs based largely on coursework, enhanced further by knowledge based on reading and experience. In addition Christopher did not feel that at his age he wished to wait a further year before undertaking the studies he had set his heart on.

CAREER CHOICE OF MIDWIFERY

Tina is now 23, and arrived in England with her parents from Ghana when she was five years old. She left school in North London at 16, having attempted seven GCSEs, including maths and English language, but she passed only one, drama, at grade C. Moving on to further education college locally, with the support of her parents, she retook English GCSE and gained a C grade. With her confidence largely restored she took part in full-time studies, achieving a Merit profile at Intermediate, and then at Advanced GNVQ, in Health and Social Care. Within this programme, she passed mathematics as a core subject, and also took an A/S GCE-level in biology, for which she gained a D grade (pass). The programme was planned individually for Tina by the tutors and agreed by Tina, who was at that time beginning to focus on a career in health care, possibly nursing, but perhaps midwifery.

As the career decision was not resolved in her mind at that time she took the advice of the local careers service as well as guidance from her college tutors, and applied through UCAS Clearing as a late applicant for a joint honours degree programme in Health Studies with Psychology, thus keeping all her options open, but not wasting time as she developed her career. She also managed during this period of full-time study to work part time some evenings of the week as a supermarket check-out cashier, still living at home with her family.

During the final year of her honours degree Tina became confirmed in her wish to become a midwife, partly based on visits to hospital placements, but mainly on her involvement with her sister's pregnancy and delivery within her close family. She researched her options through the UCAS web pages, and applied through UCAS/NMAS in the normal application cycle and deadlines, to be able to give her the best chances of attaining her first choice of university and hospitals. The UCAS/NMAS application form for the Diploma in Midwifery gave her four choices within her region. Tina needs to gain an NHS bursary for the next stages of her education, as she has already had a student loan for her earlier degree studies.

It is likely that she will be awarded a bursary when she gains her place on the Midwifery Diploma programme, for which she is ready, well prepared and now firmly committed to. She has become a very good candidate, now that she has improved her entry qualifications, but more particularly since she can demonstrate a maturity and commitment in her ultimate career choice.

CAREER CHOICE IN PRIMARY HEALTH
NEW DEVELOPMENTS AND RESEARCH

Jackie is already a Registered Nurse, qualifying as an RGN in 1985. Since this time she has worked in nursing as a staff nurse in a hospital that is accredited for education and training of nurses, graduate doctors and other health professionals, although it is not a so-called teaching hospital undertaking undergraduate medical training and education.

Jackie was promoted to ward sister of a mixed men's and women's surgical ward at an early age, and took responsibility for the management of the ward, its teams of nursing staff and the ultimate overseeing of the care given to patients within her charge. Another aspect of job satisfaction at this time was working in multiprofessional teams together with the surgical and anaesthetic teams of doctors who had performed the operations.

Jackie has now moved on, having married a local general practitioner, and assisted in the practice where there were four other doctors and three practice nurses. The change of emphasis of patient care towards care in the community, together with the knowledge of GP fund holding, GPs' increasing role in a series of minor operations, and day-case surgery, has spurred Jackie into considering her own career path with further options. Although she has gained substantial experience, which is documented in the Professional Portfolio she is obliged to keep as a practising nurse, she is aware that she now needs to undertake more formal development and training in order to fulfil her career role as a nurse, and no doubt informally to improve her own job satisfaction.

With her RGN Jackie was credited with 120 general credits towards degree or diploma studies. As she is already registered as a nurse she feels that a degree programme is her next move, probably undertaken part time because of her family commitments. In discussion with two universities near to her home, she verified where she might be admitted to the programmes with advanced standing at interview. Jackie was able to apply to both of these universities as a direct applicant, without going through UCAS, as she was expecting to study for an undergraduate degree part time.

Although ambitious to get through these studies quickly, and therefore start on the programmes with as much credit towards the degree as possible, with the help of the university tutors Jackie realised that she should not be placed too far along the programme without sufficient underpinning of earlier foundation studies. In Jackie's case this amounted to doing two foundation modules, one in information technology and the other in the support module on research methods, in which she wanted ultimately to score highly as it was a central module for the overall programme.

31

Her joint honours degree programme choice was Health Studies with Business Studies, with the underlying reason that she would ultimately like to work in full-time research, possibly for the King's Fund for London or a similar organisation at national or international level. If she does not achieve this particular goal she has a further and equally worthwhile reason underpinning her degree choice: as an experienced health professional well versed in unit management, she has a lot to offer and explore in the world of primary health care, GP fund holding and practice management, where much, including GP tasks, is changing, especially with day-case surgery and minor operations performed in the health centre itself.

Jackie has a talent for being ahead of what is needed in nursing services. It is difficult to predict what she will finally achieve, but at the present time it looks as if she will be at the forefront of future changes in nursing developments. Jackie may have to consider whether she wishes to undertake nurse development with accelerated programmes to become a medical practitioner, which at the time of going to press is under consideration in some university training partnerships.

NEW AND SECOND CAREER CHOICE AS NURSING ASSISTANT

Jo left school at 18 with seven GCSEs, including maths and English language, and two A-level GCEs in design and theatre studies, both with grade EE. Declining to study further at that time, she had several exciting jobs in the clothes industry, as trainee buyer or retailer, finally developing herself within management training in personnel. She holds qualifications by part-time study, in work-based study programmes both at undergraduate diploma and postgraduate level, but at no time has she entered studies for an undergraduate degree.

Jo married at a relatively young age and has had two children who are now both starting school. As a bright and personable young mother with time to offer, and sufficient experience with people, she wishes to offer these skills again, both within her own current context but also with an eye to a future career if things pan out that way.

Sensibly Jo addressed this problem as she saw it, by looking in the jobs columns of the local newspapers, where she noticed some regular advertising for nursing assistants who could work the shifts and hours that were suitable to them through a banking arrangement via a local agency.

Following several long telephone calls and discussions Jo finally found the confidence to apply to become a nursing assistant at the local community hospital, allowing her to undertake night shifts whilst her husband put the children to bed, arriving back for breakfast and to take the children to school in the village.

The full-time, trained staff have trained Jo for the basic tasks that she has to fulfil, including assisting with care of post-operative patients and older people with medical conditions as well as those with cancer needing respite care. Her early and first training involved learning how to lift patients properly without injury to either herself or the patient. She is always part of a team, and knows that the tasks she is undertaking are part of a nurse's duties allocated to her so that the fully trained nurse may get on with other, more difficult tasks. This is part of the assessment of the skill mix needed to undertake any nursing task, and may assist in the better use of team time. Jo feels that because of this she now has a worthwhile job, with hours that are agreed by her, working with people who need her assistance using her own skills as a caring human being as well as a nursing assistant. The pay is hourly and relatively low, hardly a wage to live on, but as a part-time job with other support it is acceptable.

Jo expects to undertake NVQ assessments of the tasks that she does, and ultimately may choose to enter nursing more fully by this route. Which branch and which speciality may be difficult for her to determine at this time. Watch this space!

CAREER CHOICE OF WARD SISTER IN MIDWIFERY

Anita was doubly qualified and registered both as a general nurse and as a midwife after finishing her studies in 1990. She came to Britain from Mauritius to undertake these studies, having taken six O-levels at school, leaving at 17. She started her general registration training at 17½, in Mauritius, and studied in Cambridge for her midwifery registration.

After her first appointment as a staff nurse in midwifery she applied to UCAS as a late applicant for a joint honours programme in Nursing and Midwifery Studies. Although her studies were full time she managed to work hours by arrangement for just two hospitals on a regular basis, even though she worked through an agency as a bank nurse. Anita achieved this level of support from both her hospitals and her official employer, the agency operating the bank.

Whilst studying and developing her up-to-date knowledge, both in theory and practice, her third year of study became even more pressurised as she met and married an engineer and manager. Nonetheless Anita achieved an upper second class degree by continuing to work as a midwife but finishing her modular degree studies on a flexible part-time basis. Currently Anita is a ward sister on a midwifery unit in a busy district hospital that is accredited for further training of midwives and children's nurses.

Her interests lie in the sustained work done with the home-from-home delivery of babies and in enhancing the work done by midwives before, during and after labour in the community setting. She does not feel that the hospital ward is either a pinnacle of practice or an area working in isolation from the community.

CAREER CHOICE OF NEW NURSING DEVELOPMENTS AND PRACTICE/NHS CALL DIRECT

Jennie, now 25, undertook an honours degree in Nursing and qualified to practice (registration) just three years ago. The challenge of understanding the biological and social sciences that underpin and inform nursing practice are sometimes daunting, especially as they are taught first within the degree or diploma programmes, even though this is alongside nursing theory and practice.

Jennie always felt that the degree programmes were the start of new thinking about people's health, and allowed her to challenge her own traditional beliefs as to whose health it is anyway. Further, these approaches led her to reappraise the sort of nursing she wished to undertake, or the nurse she should become.

Autonomy and independence, modernity and challenge stimulated her to apply for a post within the new NHS Call Direct service, recently implemented in order to allow patients or clients to access personal health advice by telephone from a nurse who will respond to the enquiries by access to computer databases to support their guidance, telephone diagnostic and simple prescribing skills for over the counter remedies. Recent research suggests that this new approach is a significant one, and may be a break with tradition in a new, fast moving technological world possibly akin to telephone banking.

Jennie acknowledges that there may be a case for a professional person practising with both medical and nursing technology and skills, but she defends the position that the focus of a nurse is the care of the whole person, and the focus of a medical practitioner primarily one of disease diagnosis and specific treatment, in the interests of the whole person.

The medical and nursing debate will not go away easily and Jennie finds it both exhilarating and perplexing to be involved in this debate.

CAREER CHOICE COMMUNITY NURSING, HEALTH VISITING

Sinead is the daughter of a health visitor, but she has always purposefully away from the possibility that she herself might eventually follow in her mother's footsteps.

Sinead sees that her mother used to work with young mothers with newbo babies on their return from hospital to their own homes, sometimes along the midwife, until formal patient handover, as part of community team ca Now her mother works with older clients in health surveillance and gives advice on healthy living as she herself relates to older people well and is received by them for advice and assistance.

Sinead has already started on a single honours degree programme in Sociology, but found that the subjects she felt most comfortable with wer those concerned with health or sociology related to government policy. S feels that she is now not able to undertake further studies as financially s limited in her options.

However, when visiting the careers advice centre of her university and c talking with her mother, she has discovered that she could gain an NHS bursary in order to undertake a programme leading to registration in chi nursing, adult nursing or community nursing. Following this advice, her step was to research the available programmes and locations through th UCAS web page.

Sinead's next worries involved whether she would be personally suited style of life and work, so she did several weeks of role-shadow in the s vacation just to check this out for herself, mainly to prove whether she the necessary patience, tolerance and people skills. This has proved ve useful in completing the application form for entry to the first part of tl Nursing Register. The second part of Sinead's commitment will be to e specialist programmes leading to health visiting practice, but at least sl knows where she is going and has started on the road.

Chapter 5
WHAT DO I HAVE TO OFFER, AND WHAT SHOULD I STUDY BEFORE I APPLY?

Personal reflection should be able to confirm for you that you are making an informed choice in your next steps in your life and your career path. You need to take sufficient time to make this choice. No one can tell you how much time is enough. Do not make your decision until you have spent some considerable time gathering information, and then pause to reflect that this is what you want to do.

The next part of the process needs you to analyse whether this is a realistic choice, given that we all have strengths and weaknesses. Sometimes your passion to become a nurse or midwife may have overruled aspects of your life, your personality and your needs that demand consideration. Take time for reflection again.

It would be neither kind nor appropriate if the following tough words were left out of this or any other advisory book on how to apply for nursing or another caring profession.

There are some individuals who are excluded or discouraged from entering nurse or midwifery education. For example, someone who has a history of mental illness will probably not, in the long term, be able to survive the intensive self-assessment and rigorous education process demanded by nursing. It is very important that you do not refuse to acknowledge past mental illness. You will not be of any benefit to yourself, or to your patients or clients if you do. If you have such a history but are well enough to undertake undergraduate studies, then

discuss your options with some care with a qualified careers officer or teacher working in careers guidance. You may be advised to apply for non-clinical degree studies related to social studies or health studies, which may broaden your choices.

The second area concerns any individual with a past history of serious criminal offending. A police check for such records is performed on all applicants to nursing and social service careers that provide care to vulnerable people. If the applicant to nursing is below the age of 18 (the minimum age for entrance is 17½ years) then a parent will normally be asked for consent.

Now for the positive side. You have no doubt got much to offer in terms of a career in nursing or midwifery, so let's explore the potential.

Your strengths

Why not list these? They may include:

- your disposition and people skills
- your academic achievement
- your sense of humour
- your outside interests, travels and occupations, if appropriate
- the levels and length of any earlier work or experience, in caring, with older people, with children, either in your family or in a care home
- your inner strengths, eg your ability to cope with long hours, or loyalty tested in difficult times.

There are many other personal attributes of this nature that you may like to discuss with your career advisers.

Your weaknesses

Be honest in your assessment. List your weaknesses and then work on any strategies to acknowledge them, and then to minimise them.

If you think any are serious enough to interfere with your ability either to study at this level, or to become a professional nurse, then talk this through with the careers advisers or teachers involved with career information. Do not leave these thoughts undiscussed, as there may be ways in which these problems can be resolved given time and sound advice from professional career advisers.

More positively you might also test out your worries by undertaking an Access to Nursing programme at your local college of further education. A decision not to enter a course leading to nursing or midwifery might be the right one for you at this time.

WHAT SHOULD I STUDY BEFORE I APPLY TO COLLEGE OR UNIVERSITY?

It is important to recognise that you will be expected to work at the level of higher education during your nursing and midwifery studies in a university, or college of higher education, and during your clinical studies in hospital or the community.

Nurse assistant

If you know that this is too high a level for you to work at this time, and you know that you still wish to nurse in an assistant, non-registered role, then you should contact your local hospital for employment as a nursing assistant. You may possibly enter the register at a later date, through some of the vocational studies qualifications that you will probably achieve whilst working, and being assessed through your workplace. The most important thing to remember is that life is a journey of studies, lifelong learning, and it is expected of us all that we continue to study and learn new skills throughout our lives, to respond to the constant demand of change. (See Jo, in the case studies in Chapter 4.)

Mature applicant

If you are a mature applicant by definition (ie over 21 years old) there are still some prerequirements to be met in terms of statutory academic qualifications before you may enter nursing and midwifery studies, ie before you are eligible to enter, even though you may not need the standard form of entry requirements for higher education as those going direct from school or further education college.

Mature students may enter higher education without formal qualifications, but for entry to nursing need to demonstrate prior and recent learning within five subject areas, or the equivalent validated study. This may sometimes be achieved by completing a year studying on an Access to Nursing course. Arrangements may be made by some colleges and institutes of higher education to allow prospective students to present earlier learning experiences and formal certificated learning for accreditation of prior and experiential learning (APEL).

Mature students may also take a UKCC-validated DC Test at a single sitting. It is equivalent to taking five GCSEs, including general knowledge, all at the same time. It is not an easy option. There was a move to phase out this test, but there is still a need for a test of this nature, and it probably needs to be reappraised in some way for the future.

The applications office of the university to which you apply will advise you where you may sit this test. There are several centres that will conduct these in formal examination style and sittings. (See the profile of Christopher in Chapter 4.)

Academic qualifications for entry into particular programmes, quoted in the colleges' or universities' prospectuses, act largely as a guide, in order for you to be able to succeed in your studies, and in the particular institution you have chosen. However as people mature they gain experience, other skills and knowledge, both certificated and informal uncertificated. These aptitudes are identified at interview if you are by definition a mature student. Other attributes of your personality and skills will also be taken into account at that time. Brian Heap, in *Degree Course Offers*, discusses various courses for nursing studies and midwifery, and notes that admission requirements for nursing vary from 20 points at A-level (BCC or BB) down to four points (EE). Further research, based on UCAS annual reports, has shown that the average score on entry to nursing degree studies, which is not the same as on application, is 12 points (ie CC).

These differences between admission requirements and entry scores reflect less on the quality of various courses and more on their popularity, ie more popular courses will set higher admission requirements. They also show that A-level scores are only one indicator of aptitude for entry to professional studies at degree level. There is usually a great deal more emphasis placed on an applicant's personal qualities such as communication skills and problem solving.

In the 2002 applications cycle, the UCAS tariff, together with implementation of the new school vocational curriculum, will alter the relatively limited A-level profile available for higher education application assessment.

It is probably self-evident that you must gain a realistic appraisal of what points or profile scores you are likely to achieve to be able to choose your university and college courses with the likelihood of being admitted to one on which you can study happily and successfully.

Which subjects?

It is a good idea to aim for a broad base of subjects in your post-16 education rather than narrowing your options down to subjects similar to those you will be studying in your first year at university or college. However some preparation for some parts of the course will no doubt help, and may be an entry requirement in some instances.

Almost all the courses in most institutions are moving towards a stronger scientific emphasis, to accommodate the requirements of nursing and midwifery today and for the future. Courses usually have a prerequisite of biology and mathematics to at least GCSE pass standard. Each prospectus should state the precise requirements. If the entry requirements are not made clear in the official prospectus you should write to the university admissions office to seek formal clarification.

Your knowledge of physics and chemistry may be challenged by new subjects such as pharmacology for prescribing, therefore these subjects could be studied at GCSE level or pre-16 if available. It is possible to study sociology or psychology to A-level. These subjects are often taken by adults returning to study. However you will study social sciences throughout your course, via the topics concerning the individual, the family and society. Therefore you should choose subjects for pre-entry studies that you are good at, which interest you and that you enjoy, and that suit your particular aptitudes.

You should note, however, that not all courses accept general studies as part of their profile criteria for admission. Check carefully in the relevant prospectus, and if you are still in doubt write to the admissions office of the institution for formal clarification.

Work experience

One fundamental part of your preparation, before you write your application, is that you should have had some experience of either working or work-shadowing in the caring sector. It is always an advantage to have had some work experience in the particular area that you have identified for your career path but, whilst this is desirable, it is not essential. For example, you may wish to become a community nurse, but have not yet had the chance to spend time attached to a nurse working in the community. However you may have had experience working part-time in a residential care home. This is still valid work experience. Besides, you may change your mind about your chosen career path during the course of your studies.

THE WHOLE PERSON

Above all it is important that you enjoy your pre-university/college studies, as well as your undergraduate studies. This may be the last opportunity to indulge yourself in a subject area such as music or art.

There may be opportunities in music or art therapy later on in your career that may relate to these subjects and in which you may wish to take the option of further study and development. It would therefore be a pity if you had dropped these subjects that you enjoy, mistakenly believing that you should be concentrating only on subjects related to nursing or midwifery.

Many individuals when changing from one setting to another, as in school to university, or working life to that of student, fail to build in some form of exercise or sport for pleasure or relaxation on a regular basis. As a prospective nurse or midwife you will be seen as a role model, especially with reference to the increasing role of health education and the policy targets for a healthier nation. It would be to your credit if you could demonstrate your earlier involvement in health and exercise or sport, and continue to build it into your new lifestyle.

In summary therefore you need to spend time on reflection, as well as time on the right set of subjects for pre-entry study, and you need to spend time developing your whole person, as time invested here will be of considerable assistance to you at interview and in your future life.

Chapter 6
NECESSARY PERSONAL ATTRIBUTES FOR A CAREER AS A NURSE OR MIDWIFE

The personal attributes that you need to be a successful applicant to a nursing and midwifery degree or diploma course are those you need to be a nurse or midwife.

Clearly Project 2000 was designed and put in place for nurses and midwives of the future to gain a wide education by being full-time students in higher education, experiencing practice and relating it to underlying and related theory in nursing and midwifery studies, together with the social and life sciences.

You will be joining a profession as a student member of the team, and later, as part of that team, you will take part in rostered service during the last year of the course. Patients and members of the public will see you as a member of the nursing profession, whether you are on the first day of your course or fully qualified.

You will need to like working with people, and through this attribute be able to work more effectively with patients and clients, and also with other members of the health care team. You will need to know this for yourself and you will need to have tested this out for yourself, by working in a caring capacity for a period of time. This will demonstrate to others, your tutors and referees, that you can work effectively as part of a team to care for sick or frail people, mothers and babies, children, or those with disability.

Other less obvious attributes will become clear once you focus on the professional role that you will take up, such as the good health role model, and the ability to run your life in a health-conscious way.

Your knowledge of health education issues will be explored at interview. More importantly, you will be able to demonstrate your attitudes – to yourself, to others around you, and to those in your care.

From the start of your professional journey as a nurse or midwife you can do no better when exploring the attitudes and aptitudes needed than to consider the wider implications of the UKCC Code of Professional Conduct. Clearly the attributes of personal responsibility and the ability to reflect on personal development do not occur instantaneously. However they are central to the whole character of the person, the student nurse or midwife, the ultimate professional, and his or her professional life and practice.

The Code of Professional Conduct will underline for you the attributes needed at the time a student nurse or midwife enters clinical observation and practice, latterly as part of the rostered workforce in clinical education.

In essence, it is central to your future as a nurse or midwife that:

■ you are totally trustworthy
■ people have confidence in you
■ you are caring of others
■ you respect any information they may give you as confidential
■ you are protective of the good standing of the nursing profession and society in general
■ you are accountable for your actions and practice
■ you safeguard the well-being of any persons within your care and you are aware of issues that concern their safety
■ you can work in a team, respecting the quality of contribution from other members of that team, and above all respect the customs, values and spiritual beliefs that others may hold, and their right to hold them.

Chapter 7
HOW WILL THESE PERSONAL ATTRIBUTES BE ASSESSED?

Do not panic, this is all relatively painless, frequently fun, and sometimes pleasurably reassuring. If you really do not have these core attributes, or embryo personality profile, it is far better to find out now than waste time and effort in trying to fit yourself into the wrong mould. It would be painful to pursue the wrong path, and it is often difficult to retrace your tracks to start in the right profession or job at a later date. But even this latter course of action is better than staying on the wrong path.

1. Before you apply, do some informal self-assessment.

If you have not already done so, and you are at the stage of considering whether nursing or midwifery may be the suitable career choice for you, there are commercial interactive software programs available that assess you, your personality, your choices, likes, dislikes and aptitudes from a substantial series of answers you give to carefully framed questions.

Once you have identified the career direction in which you wish to proceed, and for which realistically you are suited, you may wish to search for specific courses at specific institutions, and this may be done using the UCAS web site, primarily for the latest information on all the undergraduate degree programmes in the UK, and ECCTIS services, a further government-supported computerised information service covering wider courses including those at Masters level.

If you do not have immediate access to the Internet yourself, then contact your local school, college, careers office, or training access point. There are over 4000 access points in the UK and British Council offices worldwide. You can use the computer yourself or with the help of an adviser. ECCTIS can also provide data for credit transfer for applicants with advanced standing and also for those who are exploring career opportunities at postgraduate level (see Chapter 4). Careers guidance at your present school or college is usually invaluable in terms of your personal assessment, as your teachers and tutors will have got to know you over a period of time, and in addition may have access to simple personality tests and questionnaires which you may like to use.

For the mature applicant, the careers centres found in most large towns, and run in conjunction with the local education authority, are an excellent source of expertise and careers counselling. The advisers there will not have had the opportunity to get to know you well, but they do have access to a range of careers guidance material.

2. The first level of formal assessment is the self-assessment required when you complete the section about yourself, your background, aspirations and achievements on your UCAS application form. You may download the form from the UCAS web site. The self-assessment section is a very important part of the form. It is probably a good idea to make a draft – or several! – before you commit yourself on the form itself. You must complete the form in your own handwriting and, because it needs to be photocopied, you need to use a black pen.

In this section you have the opportunity to let the admissions tutor know a great deal more about you, your ideas, and your writing skills. It is particularly important that you focus on why you feel that you wish to study nursing or midwifery, why you want to enter a particular course or career path and discuss why you feel that you are suited to do this, including information about your health, your wider interests and achievements, with previous experience of caring.

3. The second level of formal assessment is that done by your referees as part of the application form. Again remember, you may download the form from the UCAS web site.

A reference in this context is not to be confused with referee, as on most occasions what is written ultimately by one person about you, and on your behalf, is usually a summary of many teachers' assessments of you and your work. The exception occurs with direct entry of mature applicants, who have not first gone through an Access to Nursing course, when a single referee writes the reference.

The referee/s will have formed an opinion of you in relation to the profession you wish to join. They may know that you have spent time working in a caring capacity. It is important that they have this information about you, where you worked and for how long. It may also be helpful for them to have a written reference from someone who knows your capabilities in this area as well. The referee/s will probably have to supply an assessment of your educational ability, and your likely potential for development in higher education. All nursing and midwifery professional education now takes place either within or in close partnership with a university or college of higher education.

4. The third level of assessment is at interview.

After the application, the next assessment of your personal attributes (knowledge, skills and attitudes) is at the interview.

Your general appearance, demeanour and body language will convey and possibly reinforce many of your personal attributes during conversations at the formal interview (see Chapter 15). Do not worry if you are nervous. This is a normal reaction, and admissions tutors are used to meeting and interviewing candidates who are new to the interview process, and make allowances for a few nerves in these circumstances. In addition to the formal interview, there is informal interaction with others who are likely to have been invited for interview at the same time.

You may be shown the library or other university/hospital facilities as a group, or you may be invited to have a shared discussion on a topic such as 'Should nurses wear uniforms?' Your interaction with other potential team members, or course members, will be relevant. In other words, very simply, how do you get on with other people, and how do they relate to you?

Another more structured method, and neither better nor worse than the other methods of observational assessment discussed previously, is for you to take a simple question-and-answer short written test, or a multiple choice test. Some are known as psychometric tests, and are often used to assess a person's psychological profile and personality, and his or her potential to fulfil a particular kind of job. The psychometric tests are never used as a single assessment, but always as a portfolio of tests by which assessment will finally be made. They will only be used to endorse what is already known from your earlier profiles, and from your interview.

Alternatively you may be asked to write a single 40-minute essay on a particular topic related to the caring professions, and where you may be expected to have a well-reasoned view. The topic may be a serious one, such as 'Should euthanasia be legalised for the frail older person after living for years in a nursing home?' From this sort of question it would be possible for admissions tutors to pick out some of the qualities and attitudes of the applicant. This more sophisticated approach is frequently used for post-registration education entry, for example, or community nursing.

Whatever the framework or programme of the interview day, you will normally be given an idea of what is expected of you, including any written components. You may need to take a pen with you.

The best part of the interview day is meeting a group of like-minded people. It is even more pleasant to meet some of them again on the first day of the course.

Chapter 8
SOME NOTES ON HIGHER EDUCATION

Higher education usually takes place within a university, but it can also take place in many other institutions, such as a college or institute of higher education, or a university hospital.

The studies accomplished in these institutes may be validated to receive a degree from a nearby university, may stand alone, or may be in partnership with a university. A strand of higher education may also be achieved within a local further education college, by franchising the first year of a degree course or validating an Access course before starting degree work. The student may then finish the second and third years of the degree or diploma at the university itself, or move to the university for the full three years of the degree after completing the Access course.

For nursing and midwifery, honours degree and diploma courses in higher education are almost exclusively placed in the new universities and colleges of higher education. The degree largely grew up in the new universities because of their ability to respond quickly and sensitively to the changing professional needs of nursing and midwifery, and because they have the administrative machinery to respond more swiftly than the older universities. Some notable exceptions exist, particularly Manchester University, which developed one of the earliest degrees in nursing.

LEVELS OF STUDY

There are a number of new phrases in higher education that may need explanation.

The concept of a level of study in undergraduate degree and diploma studies is a very helpful device to allow people to study in an orderly progression, ie Level 1 progressing to Level 2, to Level 3 to graduate. It also assists people in being able to transfer the work they have achieved in one university to another. The study achieved will be given credit (accreditation) by the institution that the student is moving to, by accreditation of prior learning (APL) for the course they will be joining.

Level 1 is frequently subdivided into lA (introduction to the subject), and often incorporates 'key skills', and lB (foundation in the subject). Level 2 is defined as extension of knowledge, and Level 3 is defined as using analysis within these extended studies.

Level 4 denotes study at Masters level, which conveys a level of authority within the subject. Some of you who read for an undergraduate degree will eventually undertake Masters-level studies and read for an MSc or MA, in the process of lifelong learning.

Nursing and midwifery degrees are divided into defined parts of study, called modules. Most degrees in the UK are now modularised, ie they have defined blocks of study, with assessments at the end of each, instead of end-of-year examinations to assess all the areas of study.

Most universities and colleges follow the traditional academic arrangement of three ten-week terms a year. Recently a number of universities have introduced two 15-week semesters. However traditional Christmas and Easter breaks are incorporated into this schedule. The number of modules you will be expected to cover each week and each term or semester will vary. You should check your prospectus for these details.

The vacations are by no means 'study-free time'. In nursing you will find that you may be pursuing you studies in a variety of ways, including gaining further clinical experience. This allows you to fulfil the requirements of hours of study, both theory and clinical, laid down by the professional bodies, notably the English National Board for Nursing,

Midwifery and Health Visiting, in order to qualify and to complete the degree and diploma studies. You will also spend your vacations undertaking research projects or attending summer schools.

The undergraduate diploma (DipHE) comprises Levels 1 and 2, with some work at Level 3 on some courses. Nursing degrees comprise work at Levels 1, 2 and 3. Each level of study is completed by achieving 120 credits, and thus a further 120 credits at Levels 2/3 are required to achieve the diploma, and 360 total credits for an honours degree. It is possible to achieve a DipHE at one institution and apply through UCAS to join another to develop your studies to honours degree level. Further information on this can be found in Chapter 16. If you wish to study a particular combination of subjects at this level you are advised to visit the UCAS web site for your opportunities and choices.

ACCREDITATION OF PRIOR LEARNING

The main idea behind the modularisation and credit rating of modules of study is to be able to bank or transfer the 'credit' of successfully completed modules. These may then be used, if they are appropriate, in later studies, either at the same or another institution. Credit gained can be accumulated as 'general credit' but, when offered to gain a place on a specific, named course, the credit points have to be appropriate, and are converted into specific credit for that particular course.

It is no help at all if you enter a course with sufficient general credits but without sufficient prior development and learning to be able to be successful at the next stage. Tutors in the new institution will review what you have achieved by general credit and give you specific credit to enable you to enter your chosen course with some advanced standing.

Students who achieve 240 general credit points at Levels 1 and 2 and who successfully complete a DipHE may apply to have their general credits converted into specific credits and apply to develop their studies towards an honours degree.

A Registered General Nurse or midwife qualifying after 1985, and before the changes introduced with Project 2000 were fully implemented, can offer 120 general credit points at Level 1, toward specific credit for an honours degree course. The degree to be undertaken may or may not be in midwifery, nursing or health studies, but could be in a wider people-based study area such as social sciences, or a single subject in one of the social sciences, such as psychology, social policy, or a health-related area such as human resource management.

Specific credit in these circumstances is likely to be less than the general credit, and a foundation module in the new subject may be needed.

The decision on the amount of specific credit awarded and entry with advanced standing is always the responsibility of the receiving institution. Applications for undergraduate degrees are always through UCAS, whether advanced standing is granted or not. APL is an extremely flexible system, supporting the continuing studies of the lifelong learner.

Chapter 9
THE EFFECT OF NHS POLICY CHANGES ON GETTING INTO NURSING AND MIDWIFERY

The United Kingdom is currently divided up into 'regions' for organisational and human resource planning purposes for the National Health Service. Each of these regions is responsible for planning future workforce numbers, and thereby the numbers of nurses, midwives and other health professionals who need to be educated in order to fulfil the future needs of the region.

The region is largely responsible for purchasing the education and training that you and others will gain in order to qualify as a nurse or a midwife, health visitor or community nurse. The planning for provision of nurse professional education is achieved by partnerships with local universities and colleges of higher (or sometimes further) education.

The regional organisation in England, Wales, Scotland and Northern Ireland is responsible for the variation in the number of educational places available in each region. Education and clinical training places are limited in number, and are fixed by complex agreements at both national and local levels. Once these places are allocated no more people may join that particular course for that intake year.

It is important to have some overview of the nature of the organisation in which you are seeking a place, and in which you are most likely to be working for a substantial part of your life. The National Health Service has recently undergone a number of policy changes, undertaken largely to make the best use of future resources in an environment of growing demand. It will be useful to focus on these reforms and new structures within the health service, in order to be able to discuss these areas at interview.

Health care provision is now delivered by self-governing trusts, units of organisational activity, governed by trust boards of management, reflecting local interests as well as specialist interests. The trusts are monitored in their activities by government but are responsible for their own finances and budgets, and may in future be responsible for setting their own pay structures, inside national guidelines, including that of the nurses and midwives whom they employ. The old style district and regional health authorities have been reduced in terms of both people and powers, at the same time as the trusts have taken up their largely self-governing roles (Taylor and Field, 1997).

The hospitals and community trusts, therefore, together with the universities and colleges of higher education, are the partners interested in the education and training of future staff and, specifically in your context, in choosing candidates for nursing and midwifery, who will be able to develop, and be developed into future professional nurses and midwives.

The style and content of the courses are planned by these partners together, and validated by education quality control systems within the universities, monitored by the professional bodies, such as the national boards for Nursing, Midwifery and Health Visiting.

The four national boards, including the English National Board (ENB) are largely involved as interested parties in the education process of professional nursing and midwifery. The United Kingdom Central Council for Nursing, Midwifery and Health Visiting is responsible for the quality of professional practice and for upholding professional standards following qualification across the four locations.

Obviously, although separate, the ENB and the UKCC have a great deal in common, as the quality of good practice is founded on the quality of the education preceding it. The ENB and other national boards, together with the UKCC, are independent of the purchasing of future employment needs, but cannot be entirely separate from it, in that they are the arbiters of professional quality by statute (law).

The recent NHS policy changes can be summarised as encouraging each part of the health service, each unit, each ward or clinic to be responsible for its own management. You may expect to find yourself in charge of such a unit one day, as a unit manager or a ward sister. The challenges can be very rewarding, following personal and professional education and development to meet the of that appointment.

'Trust me, I am a nurse' may be the voice of the future, since today's nurses are responsible for many skilled procedures previously entrusted to doctors. One example is the giving of immunisations and vaccinations to those in need, as a prophylaxis against specific infections and diseases, by practice and community nurses within community and primary health care.

More health care, both primary (as in health centres and general practices) and secondary, is being given to patients in their own homes. It was planned that 'Care in the Community' would be the major part of health provision (1991), but the numbers employed in this part of the health service have yet to reflect this aspiration (Taylor and Field, 1997). The larger number of nurses and midwives are employed in the hospital context, in hospital-managed units as in the hospital trusts. Community-based nurses and midwives are employed within a Community Care Trust, and indirectly by the district health authority. These organisations interrelate by buying care from (purchasing), and giving care to (providing) each other, in a purchaser-provider relationship. Some large GP practices can also join in purchasing care from hospital trusts as they hold their own budgets separately from the district health authority.

Much of this budgetary and financial control of the NHS started in the mid 1980s on a business/commercial style of operation, in order to gain greater efficiency and efficiency-related cost savings. However, compared with other countries in the European Union, such as France and Germany, the NHS in the UK still remains underfunded in most of its components. It is a feature of the current health service in the UK that it has had to acknowledge properly, perhaps for the first time, other provision for health care, such as the private sector, which is now openly providing beds and services to hospital trusts, as and when the need arises, on the purchaser-provider basis.

For nurses and midwives this has implications for diversity and change within the sectors. None the less, the NHS is the only means by which hands-on emergency and casualty cover is provided. Healthcare provision in the private sector is largely planned, and not on an emergency basis. This could change in future years in the UK, as an insurance-based, private care system model is available for emergency medical care from the USA.

Another distinct change has been the establishment of the NHS Call Direct service, where nurses staff the telephone call centre, giving advice about health problems using computer database assistance. They may often give advice about emergency or short-term medication, with the aid of information given by the patient matched to information available to the nurse from the computer.

Changes in the way that nurses assess patients in casualty and emergency units of hospitals (triage), may influence the way that GPs, or practice nurses, respond to assessing urgent patient care within a guaranteed time at GP practices in the near future.

Change and review are very much part of the present times. Improvements in community patient care are on the current health agenda. Today's recruits to nursing and midwifery are in for an exciting and rewarding time in their new careers.

Part 2
ESSENTIAL PREPARATIONS FOR A SUCCESSFUL OUTCOME

Chapter 10
OK, SO I STILL WANT TO BE A NURSE

The essential preparations for a successful outcome to your application must include a check-up on your current educational position, together with an honest assessment of your personal development. If you find that you do not meet the strict criteria of the entry requirements, then you may need to go back a stage or two and concentrate on achieving these before you make an application, otherwise you will clearly be disappointed by your lack of success. This could also mean that you may find yourself on the wrong course or in the wrong professional role.

CHECKLIST FOR APPLICATION CRITERIA

1. Will you be over 17½ years of age on entry to university or college of higher education?
2. Do you really know that you can work with people?
3. Have you gained evidence both for yourself and others that you can work in the care sector looking after people?
4. Is it really nursing or midwifery that interests you, or have you not yet made up your mind as to your final career path, or your professional role in caring?
5. Will you be able to study full time for at least three years within higher education (for diploma and degree courses within the model of Project 2000)?
6. Do you fulfil the minimum entry requirements for nursing or midwifery studies at the time of your application? These minimum

requirements usually differ for midwifery compared with nursing. Check these again.

7. Do you have a criminal record? This will be checked on receipt of your application.
8. Are you in good health, and do you expect to remain so?
9. Do you understand the criteria to be met in the UKCC Code of Professional Conduct?
10. Can you live by these criteria for the remainder of your professional life?

Chapter 11
APPLYING THROUGH THE SYSTEM

If you have successfully completed the checklist in Chapter 10, and have undertaken a long period of reflection, you will now have a clear idea that a career in nursing or midwifery is a real possibility rather than a hope. Your next step is to pursue your goal with purpose.

At present, you may apply through UCAS for all undergraduate degrees and diplomas in nursing and midwifery. There is one application cycle per year for entry to the institutions of higher education in late September. There are a series of timed deadlines for later applications over the year, but the major deadline for receipt of most applications is mid December for the September entry of the following year. These dates, which vary slightly each year, are available and updated on the UCAS web site, but also available from career advisers in schools and careers offices. Some course programmes have a February start. You will need to check the UCAS web site and *Handbook* for information about those institutions that allow entry to programmes at this time.

The University and Colleges Admissions Service is necessary to bring order to the applications process. The large number of institutions together with the large number of applicants, would lead to chaos if there were no central coordination of which place is offered and to whom.

APPLYING THROUGH UCAS

You may make up to six choices of institution or undergraduate degree course from the codes listed in the UCAS *Handbook* or shown on the

UCAS web site, using one form per application year, including 'Clearing', the final round of places to be gained for the year's cycle. There are some minor paperwork transactions to be completed if you are still looking for a place during Clearing, but they all follow on from your initial and only application. When your initial application has been received and processed, you will start to receive replies from your chosen institutions. Assuming you have been offered more than one place, you should accept one offer as your firm choice (Cf), and another requiring lower grades or point scores as your insurance choice (Ci). You should then decline any remaining offers.

There are many well-informed and well-written texts offering advice on what you should consider when you make these decisions. Your choices are final and therefore very important. A list of recommended texts is given at the end of this book.

If you are applying for DipHE programmes only, through the subsidiary office of the Nurses and Midwives Admissions Service (NMAS) at UCAS, intending to gain an associated bursary with the programme place, you may apply for up to four programme choices on the NMAS form, within your local NHS region. Some universities may admit you for either February or September entry for the DipHE programmes. It pays to check this out with the institutions you have chosen, and which time of the year fits your own personal plans (see Tina in the case studies in Chapter 4).

CLEARING

Applying through UCAS to a total of six institutions for a place in higher education to study for an undergraduate degree or diploma gives you a good chance of gaining a place somewhere, providing you meet the minimum entry requirements. However, if you miss out in the first and subsequent rounds of the cycle of gaining a place for the year in which the application was made, and consequently still hold no offer at all, then the number of institutions becomes much wider in the process known as 'Clearing', which occurs in mid-August, before the September start. This is a means by which the final places are filled.

To take part in Clearing, UCAS issues applicants already in the system, but holding no offers at all, a Clearing C-form to be completed in order for applicants to secure the place that they will be finally offered. This has been termed an unofficial passport to gain and confirm a place on your behalf, without which the place cannot be secured.

If you find that you do not want to accept your original choice of Cf or Ci institution, then you must formally reject the offers you have received and take your chance by entering Clearing. You cannot enter Clearing unless you have rejected all offers or you hold no offers whatever at that time. Only then will you be issued with a C-form.

Chapter 12
CHOOSING YOUR COLLEGE OR UNIVERSITY AND GETTING CHOSEN

CHOOSING

Nursing and midwifery are no longer in the unusual position that individuals are educated to professional status, and then develop to professional status in isolation in schools of nursing and midwifery, separate from other professional groups. Now, all the benefits and resources available to other higher education entrants are available to those entering nursing, midwifery and the many other health professional degree career pathways that develop from initial qualification and registration. As a consequence, all the information that is available and can be made to work for you, in addition to all the specialist information that you have concerning the education processes for nursing and midwifery, are yours for the taking.

The section about getting into university and college on the UCAS web site provides a short and highly relevant guide and checklist that allows you to take charge of your own choices leading to an undergraduate degree or diploma programme. Detail is given as to how you may make your choice; make a timetable to achieve a good outcome; consider criteria in choosing among differing courses; and the choice of institution, together with the choice of location – city, suburban or rural settings – even perhaps university sports facilities. Similarly a great deal of unofficial information is given by Brian Heap in *Degree Course Offers*, updated annually. These key references are available in most libraries or careers offices and are referenced at the end of this book.

Once you have made a shortlist of courses and locations, write to the relevant institutions and obtain any promotional literature, together with the prospectus, including the alternative prospectus produced by the Students Union, for a different view of the institution. Remember any promotional material produced by the institution is designed to show it in the most favourable light. When your shortlist is reduced to six, make every effort to visit them on open days for a closer view. A virtual tour of some of your chosen university towns and campuses may assist in making the best use of the time you have available for visits and information gathering.

GETTING CHOSEN

Your first formal contact with the institution to which you have applied will be via your application form, and this must be filled in correctly. Details on getting it right and getting it in by the stated deadlines are given in the UCAS *Handbook* and on the web site, and also in the helpful monograph, 'How to Complete Your UCAS Form [for current year] Entry'.

It may seem self-evident, but to be successful in your application for a place to study nursing or midwifery your application form must be completed accurately and posted in time to reach UCAS by the due deadline.

Make sure your referees know what is expected of them, and what areas they should cover on your behalf. This is a reference to support your entry into higher education, not a job application. Sometimes referees in the workplace do not understand this difference, nor have knowledge of you in this capacity. It is your responsibility to check this through, and not the responsibility of the receiving institution to have to write for a fuller reference if the first one does not give enough appropriate information.

What happens if several institutions make you an offer?

If this is the case, hard choices have to be made, and by a given deadline, or all offers may go by default. If time is short, do not forget to look at virtual visits to the campuses or towns, available through the UCAS web site.

Then, before your deadline, choose your designated firm offer, Cf, and your designated insurance offer, Ci, by reference to all the information you obtained earlier. The firm offer is one you hold until all the conditions of the offer are met, or not. The insurance offer is held just in case you do not make the grade requirements of your firm offer.

However the Ci must also be a realistic choice, a course or institution that you will be willing to accept if you cannot meet the requirements of your Cf.

Chapter 13
IF AT FIRST YOU DON'T SUCCEED ...

If you are not successful in your first round of applications, and you are still keen to get on a course, try Clearing. There are publications to assist your progress through Clearing, primarily *Clearing the Way* by T. Higgins (published by Trotman), which gives an information path and simple guide to assist those working their way through the UCAS clearing process, attempting to find a place on an undergraduate degree or diploma programme in nursing or midwifery in the few weeks before the start of the term or semester. The original application form generates an automatic Clearing entry form, the C-form, when the applicant has not yet gained a place and also holds no offers in the UCAS system.

The first thing to remember is not to panic and not to make rash, unconsidered decisions.

The second thing to remember is that you must be realistic. Most people who are qualified will eventually find a place within the system, but not necessarily studying the subject or at the level they first wished. This may mean that you may have to start by studying for a diploma and then work towards getting a degree, by programmes available for development to a degree at a later stage. For further information on the style, content and availability of such top-up programmes, visit the UCAS web site.

As you develop through the diploma programme that you have chosen through Clearing, you may find that the many options available to you in the top-up programmes leading to the honours degree may suit your later thinking and progress better than you expected.

Chapter 14
I AM A REGISTERED NURSE AND WISH TO STUDY FOR A DEGREE

(Refer to Anita and Jackie in the case studies in Chapter 4.)

The date of your registration is significant in this context, and in the next stages of your learning development. If you registered and qualified as a nurse or midwife after 1985 in the UK, then you have gained 120 general credit points at Level 1 in undergraduate studies. How these are translated into specific credits depends on the receiving institution at which you wish to study, and the subject areas of the degree you wish to enrol upon. The likelihood is that you may need to study for all of Levels 2 and 3, for 240 points, plus an extra module at foundation level to support your work in any new subject area, if you choose a joint honours degree in two subjects.

It is a matter of matching your past achievements to the degree programme you wish to enrol on, in order for you to be successful. It probably makes good sense for you to study for a degree rather than a diploma. as you are already qualified and on the professional register as a nurse or midwife, and can already work professionally in this context.

All full-time undergraduate degree applications are handled by UCAS, even though you may wish only to apply to a single institution, and for a single course, and the tutors have given you a verbal offer of a place. You must send for or obtain a current UCAS form, follow all the instructions in detail, including referees, fee and timing of responses. You might even wish to exercise the remainder of your six options of institutions.

Although all initial nursing and midwifery degrees and diplomas are full time, top-up or post-registration courses may be studied part time. Part-time applicants for degree courses do not at the present time have to apply via UCAS, but can apply directly to the receiving institution.

As you are already registered to practise as a nurse or midwife, then your choice of degree could easily be more wide ranging than nursing and midwifery. You could study health studies, either alone or with another closely allied subject such as psychology, sociology, women's studies, third world studies, information technology, human resource management, business or education studies. This may open up more career paths, and wider options in the NHS or other agencies, working across the globe. Check out your options among a wealth of courses available, by content and location, through the UCAS web site. Many NHS bursary programmes have substantial practical applications and these may lead on to further developments in different career paths (these can be found in the 'top-up' programmes identified on the UCAS web site).

If you registered before 1985, then you may apply for the same range of degree options but you may not gain any general or specific credit in the programme. You will enter at Level 1, and proceed through the degree programme in the usual way. Your application should be made through UCAS for a full-time course and direct to university or college for part-time study. Full-time study qualifies for student loan and fees facilities, whereas support for part-time study largely relies on personal finances, unless your employer can be persuaded to support your studies. Many GP practices and trusts do fund their employees and give them time to attend formal studies. Sometimes to assist in staff retention and development, it is part of the job package from the outset. Think about this if you are about to negotiate a new contract.

Information on the complex area of student funding and student finance is available on the UCAS web site and also through the NHS Student Grants Unit. The main message to most applicants is that you should apply for a student loan facility if you are applying for a full-time degree programme. Make no assumptions as to what you are entitled to, as you may be entitled to more support than you think. Undergraduate diploma programmes are financed by bursaries from the region to which you have applied. The finance goes with the place on the programme and is managed by the university at which you are studying.

If you are a mature applicant, defined as someone over 21 years of age, with related work or life experiences over a period of time, then you may need a more targeted form of careers advice in order to maximise your chances of gaining a place at university or college. Motivated mature students up to the age of 40 usually achieve better degree results than their younger, standard-entry counterparts.

Recommended reading should again include the advice section for the mature applicant on the UCAS web site, and further reading to assist the mature applicant is listed at the end of this book.

Part 3
NEXT STEPS IN LIFELONG LEARNING

Chapter 15
PERSONAL RECORD OF EDUCATION AND PROFESSIONAL PRACTICE (PREP)

Many nurses and midwives already in practice do not fit into any of the earlier categories of students or prospective students in lifelong learning. Yet they still need to appraise what learning they have already achieved, and to have it recognised formally, in order to build on it and to improve their clinical practice.

Clearly nursing and midwifery, as with many other professions, need to respond to major changes taking place in practice and in clinical developments and settings, as well as keep pace with major social changes in health-related matters. The national boards for Nursing, Midwifery and Health Visiting have initiated and developed a framework for collating and presenting a Personal Record of Education and Professional Practice (PREP), not unlike the student Record of Achievement used in schools. The majority of nurses and midwives in practice, 70 per cent, are reported as fulfilling their PREP requirements fully, and 86 per cent are reported as structuring their learning activity through courses. Copies of advisory documents concerning PREP are available from the UKCC and from their website.

The PREP may be used in a similar manner to the Record of Achievement. Records of continuing education for lifelong learning will be a regular feature of job applications and personal profiles. Evidence of learning achievement allows individuals to be credited with what they have done at all levels of their work and practice.

Chapter 16
I HAVE A DIPLOMA IN NURSING OR MIDWIFERY AND WISH TO STUDY FOR A DEGREE

The Diploma in Higher Education forms the main route for the education of nurses and midwives to initial registration. It forms the first two levels of the undergraduate degree, thus representing 240 general credits points for transfer. If the holder of a diploma in nursing or midwifery wishes to study for a degree, he or she should apply via UCAS if study is to be full time. Application for part-time, as opposed to full-time, top-up degree programmes should be made direct to the receiving institution.

A student loan facility may be available for study and living support, if the study is full time and you have not previously held a grant or similar support.

Most applicants who study part time on degree programmes are supported to varying levels by the trusts or others that employ them, including of course giving the midwife or nurse time off in order to attend the programme at the nearby university or university hospital. Some programmes have been undertaken in this context as distance learning. Unfortunately these have not proved to be the success story that was originally hoped for. Students have tended to drop out after the first year of such studies as many employers have not thought it necessary to give time off for study, as there was little time spent attending classes. The other problem factor was that students like to meet other students and share experiences. This support and professional interaction was not built into the early programmes involving distance learning. Professional experiences are a large component of professional development, particularly in the context of nursing, midwifery and multi-professional developments.

The variety of degree subject areas for which you may apply are wider than those in nursing and midwifery, and are described for the person who has a post-1985 RGN, in Chapter 14. Joint honours degrees widen your options and your job opportunities. Modular science-based subjects, such as pharmacology or epidemiology, may enhance your development to assist the changes taking place in nursing practice for the future. These modules are often part of a modular science-based degree in health studies, forming an Honours BSc degree, but may also form joint subject degree programmes with nursing or midwifery. The wide and diverse subjects on offer to you, both in single subject or joint subject honours can be seen by a visit to the UCAS web site.

Chapter 17
THE PROFESSIONAL BODIES

The English National Board for Nursing, Midwifery and Health Visiting (ENB), in partnership with universities and colleges, is largely responsible for the quality of professional education of nurses, midwives and health visitors in England today. It has been centrally involved in the understanding that it is the quality of education which leads to the quality of care, and it uses this phrase for its logo. There are similar boards for Wales, Northern Ireland and Scotland, defined and put in place by government statute.

Similarly, the national statutory body responsible for practice quality and accountability is the United Kingdom Central Council for Nursing, Midwifery and Health Visiting (UKCC). This body is responsible for monitoring the Code of Professional Conduct for practising nurses and midwives. This Code provides the focus for exploring and maintaining the personal qualities that are needed for practice as a nurse or midwife.

The UKCC is also responsible for disciplinary procedures if the quality of practice is not adhered to. Nurses can be removed from the Register and from practice. Education and practice standards are closely interwoven and, as a consequence, these two bodies relate to each other closely, and may become more linked in the future.

The other major player in the national forum for nursing is the Royal College of Nursing (RCN). A similar senior organisation exists for midwives (the RCM). The RCN has two main arms of operation: one functions largely as the political voice of nursing, holding talks with government and other national agencies, representing its members when and where necessary; the other arm is that of an institute of higher education and of advanced nursing education, as at the Royal College of

Nursing Institute, where postgraduate studies are achieved, for post-registration nurses and midwives who have already achieved registration through earlier studies and clinical practice.

All of these national bodies have been changing swiftly and dramatically in response to current nursing professional health changes, which they in turn have been involved in. They are the leading bodies responsible for taking nursing forward in the 21st century.

Chapter 18
RESOURCE INFORMATION AND CONTACT DATA

USEFUL ADDRESSES

Department of Health
PO Box 777
London SE1 6XH
for information leaflet, 'Financial
Help for Students'
email: doh@prologistics.co.uk

NHS Student Grants Unit
Room 212C Government Building
Norcross
Blackpool
FY5 3TA
Tel 0125 3856 123

NHS Careers (England)
PO Box 376
Bristol BS99 3EY
Tel 0845 6060 655
email: advice @nhscareers.nhs.uk
www.nhs.uk/careers

English National Board for
Nursing, Midwifery and Health
Visiting (ENB)
Victory House
Tottenham Court Road
London W1A 0XA
Tel 020 7391 6291/6305

Scotland admissions
NBS Catch
PO Box 21
Edinburgh EH2 1NT
Tel 013 1247 6622

N Ireland admissions
School of Nursing and Midwifery
Registry Office
The Queen's University of Belfast
1–3 College Park East
Belfast BT7 1LQ
Tel 028 9027 3754/9033 5116

N Ireland
National Board for Nursing, Midwifery and Health Visiting for NI
79 Chichester St
Belfast BT1 4JE
Tel 028 9023 8152
email: enqs@nbni.n-i.nhs.uk

Scotland
National Board for Nursing,
Midwifery and Health Visiting
(careers)
22 Queen Street
Edinburgh EH2 1NT

Tel 0131 225 2096
email: careers @nbs.org.uk
www.nbs.org.uk

Wales
Welsh National Board for Nursing,
Midwifery and Health Visiting
2nd Floor, Golate House
101 St Mary Street
Cardiff CF1 1DX
Tel 01222 261400
email: info@wnb.org.uk
www.wnb.org.uk

Community and District Nursing
Association
Thames Valley University
Westel House
32–38 Uxbridge Road
London W5 2BS
Tel 020 8280 5032

Institute of Health Care Management
7–10 Chandos Street
London WIM 9DE
Tel 020 7460 7654 www.ihm.org.uk

Royal College of Nursing
20 Cavendish Square
London W1M 0DB
Tel 020 7409 3333 www.rcn.org.uk

Royal College of Midwives
15 Mansfield Street
London W1M 0BE
Tel 020 7312 3535
email: info@rcm.org.uk

Unison
Mabledon House

London WC1H 9AJ
Tel 020 7388 2366

United Kingdom Central Council
for Nursing, Midwifery and Health
Visiting (UKCC)
23 Portland Place
London W1N 3AF
Tel 020 7637 7181 www.ukcc.org.uk

Universities and Colleges
Admissions Services (UCAS)
Rosehill
New Barn Lane
Cheltenham
Gloucestershire GL52 3LZ
Tel 01242 227788 www.ucas.com

Nurses and Midwives Admissions
Service (NMAS) for England
Rosehill
New Barn Lane
Cheltenham
Gloucestershire GL52 3LZ
Tel 01242 223707 www.nmas.ac.uk

Trotman Publishing
2 The Green
Richmond
Surrey TW9 1PL
Tel 020 8486 1150
www.careers-portal.co.uk

ECCTIS Ltd
Oriel House
Oriel Road
Cheltenham
Gloucestershire GL50 1XP
Tel 01242 252627 www.ectis.co.uk

BIBLIOGRAPHY

Bartlett, E and Field, M (1999) *Working as a Nurse*, How to Books.

Careers in Nursing (2000) 2nd edn, *Your Questions and Answers*, Trotman.

Dixon, B (1999) 2nd edn, *Choosing your Postgraduate Course*, Trotman.

Heap, B (2000) 31st edn, *Degree Course Offers*, Trotman.

Heap, B (2000) 7th edn, *Choosing Your Degree Course and University*, Trotman.

Higgins, T (2000) 12th edn, *Clearing the Way*, Trotman.

Higgins, T (2000) *How to complete your UCAS form for 2001 Entry*, Trotman.

Macleod Clark, J et al (1996) *Project 2000: Perceptions of the Philosophy and Practice of Nursing*, ENB.

NHS Careers literature, *Nursing and Midwifery in the new NHS*.

Nickell, H (2000) *Surfing your Career*, How to Books.

Taylor, S and Field, D (eds) (1997) 2nd edn, *Sociology of Health and Health Care*, Blackwell Science: Ch. 2 Health and health care in modern Britain; Ch. 7 Chronic illness and physical disability; Ch. 8 Mental disorders; Ch. 11 Recent trends in Health policy: consumerism and managerialism; Ch. 12 Nurses and nursing.

UCAS (1996) *A Mature Students Guide to Higher Education*, UCAS.

UCAS (2000) *University and College Entrance: The Official Guide*, UCAS.

UKCC Code of Professional Conduct, UKCC.

UKCC Midwives Rules and Code of Practice, UKCC.

UKCC (2000) *PREPP and You*, UKCC.

USEFUL WEBSITES

Trotman Careers Publishers	careers-portal.co.uk
Careers software	progressions.co.uk
Hobsons CRAC	hobsons.co.uk

Schools and College Performance Tables	dfee.gov.uk/perform.htm
Gap-year Information	thegapyear.co.uk
National Association for Special Needs	nasen.org.uk
British Dyslexia Association	bda-dyslexia.org.uk
Careers Advisory Network on Disability Options	lancs.ac.uk/staff/cpahwb/cando,htm
International Voluntary Service	ivsgbn.demon.co.uk
National Centre for Volunteering	volunteering.org.uk
The Prince's Trust	princes-trust.org.uk
Voluntary Services Overseas	vso.org.uk
Work Experience USA	workexperienceusa.com
Worldwide Volunteering	worldwidevolumteering.org.uk
Postgraduate Course Information	postgrad.hobsons.com
PUSH Guide to which universities	push.co.uk
UCAS HE Course listings	ucas.com
UK Course Discover ECCTIS	ecctis.co.uk
Health Journals listings	hjs.co.uk
British Medical Journal	bmj.com
Health Services Journal	hsj.co.uk
The Times	the-times.co.uk
Guardian newspaper	guardian.co.uk
Nursing web sites and vacancies	british-nursing.com
Royal College of Midwives Journal	midwives.co.uk
UK and European vacancies	workweb.co.uk/jobshop-co.uk
Careers Europe	careerseurope.co.uk
Graduate Employment	prospects.csu.ac.uk

NHS Careers	nhscareers.nhs.uk
English National Board for Nursing, Midwifery and Health Visiting	enb.org.uk
National Board for Nursing, Midwifery and Health Visiting in Scotland	nbs.org.uk
Welsh National Board for Nursing, Midwifery and Health Visiting	wnb.org.uk
National Board for Nursing, Midwifery and Health Visiting for N Ireland	n-i.nhs.uk/NBNI/index.htm
Royal College of Nursing	rcn.org.uk
UK Central Council for Nursing, Midwifery and Health Visiting	ukcc.org.uk
Nursing and Midwifery Admissions Service	nmas.ac.uk
Universities and Colleges Admissions Services	ucas.com
Student Choice (exams help service)	bbc.co.uk/education/choice
Student Loans Company	slc.co.uk
National Union of Students	nus.org.uk
Financial Support in Higher Education	dfee.gov.uk/support
UK Lifelong Learning	lifelonglearning.co.uk
UK and Worldwide Distance Learning Directories	distance-learning.co.uk
British Council	britcoun.org
BTEC/Edexcel (Vocational Qualifications)	edexcel.org.uk
National Vocational Qualifications	dfee.gov.uk.nvq